This book is dedicated to
my mum, who held me up
when I couldn't stand...

You can reach the author through...

Email: pitayapages@gmail.com
Instagram: @pitayapages
Ko-Fi: pitayapages

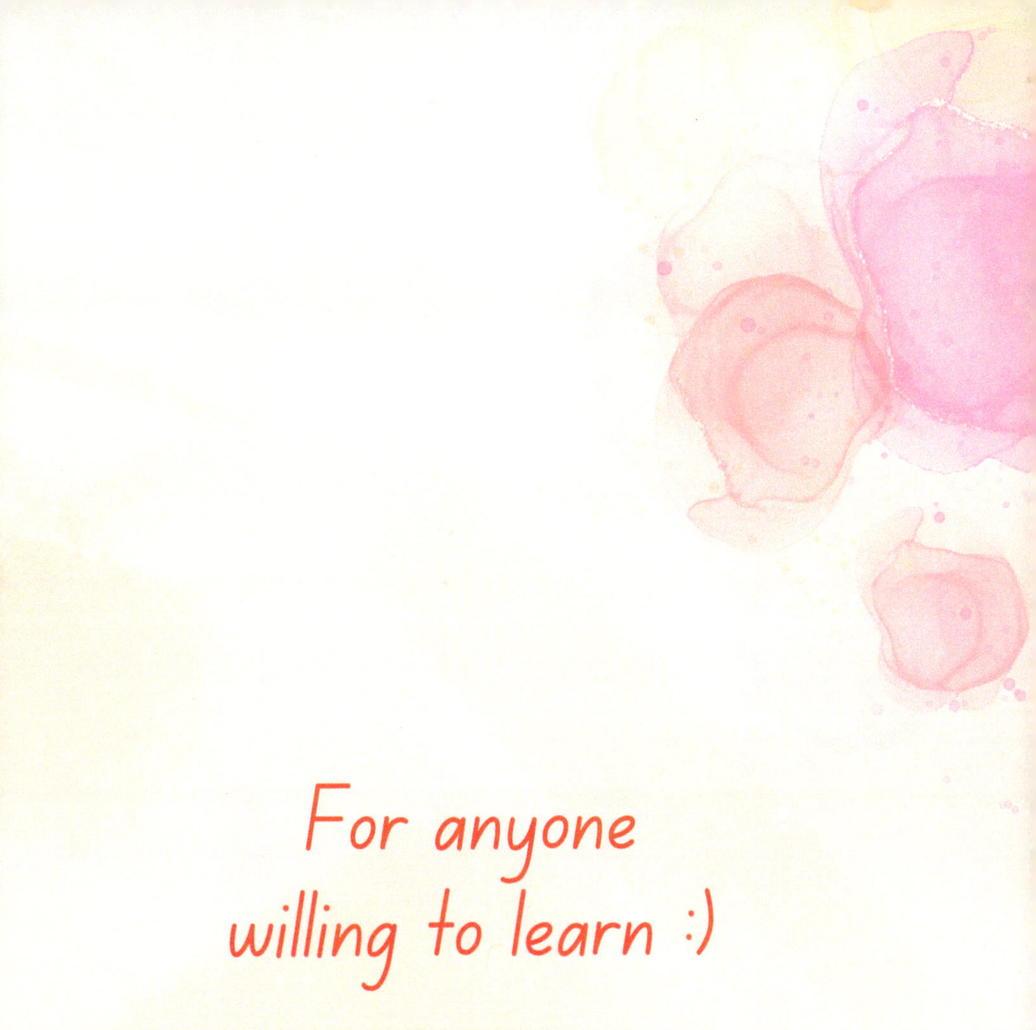

For anyone
willing to learn :)

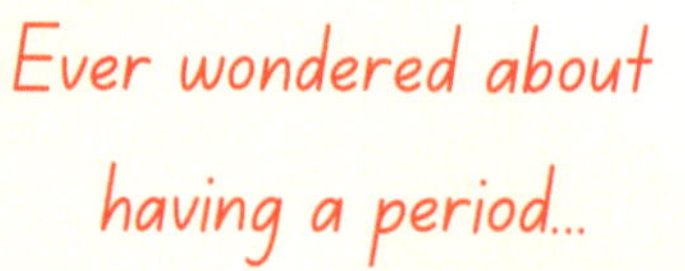

Ever wondered about
having a period...

- What are the symptoms?
- How does menstruation affect everyday life?
- How can symptoms be relieved and managed?

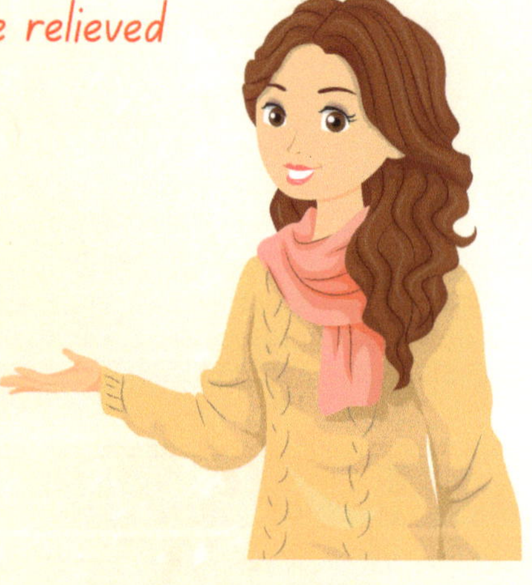

To start off, a menstrual cycle
isn't menstruation. It is the entire
hormonal pattern your body goes
through every month

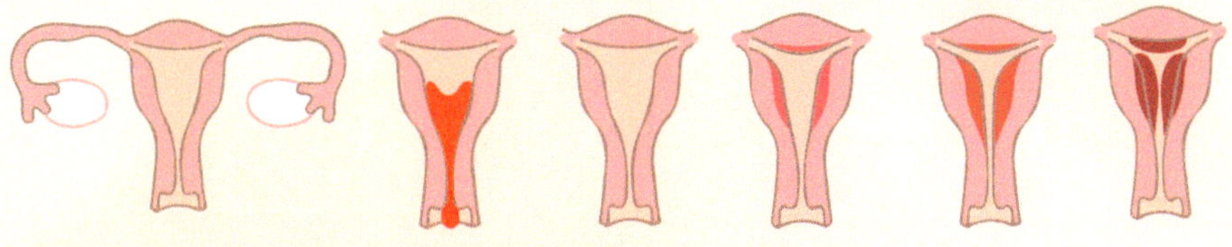

You can think of it as the
body rebooting on a loop

This is a Uterus

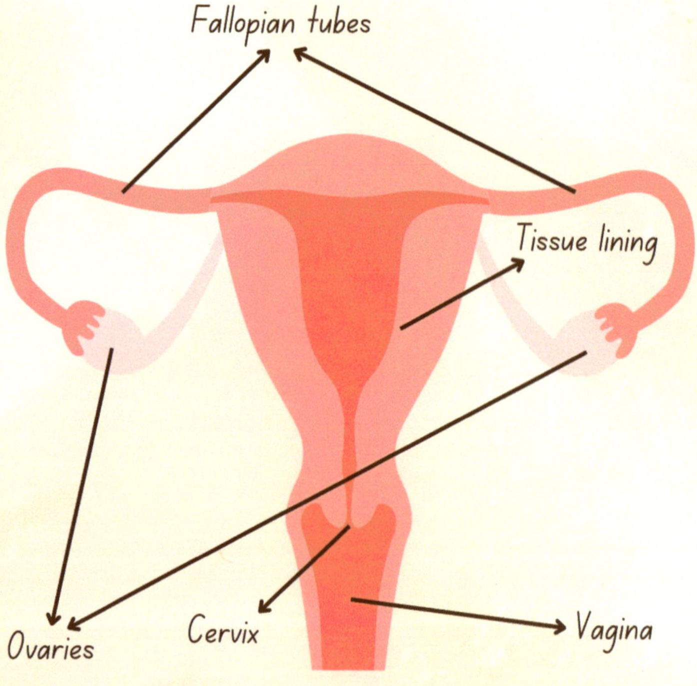

It is an organ in
the pelvic region of a
woman's body that
is responsible for
the growth and
development of a baby

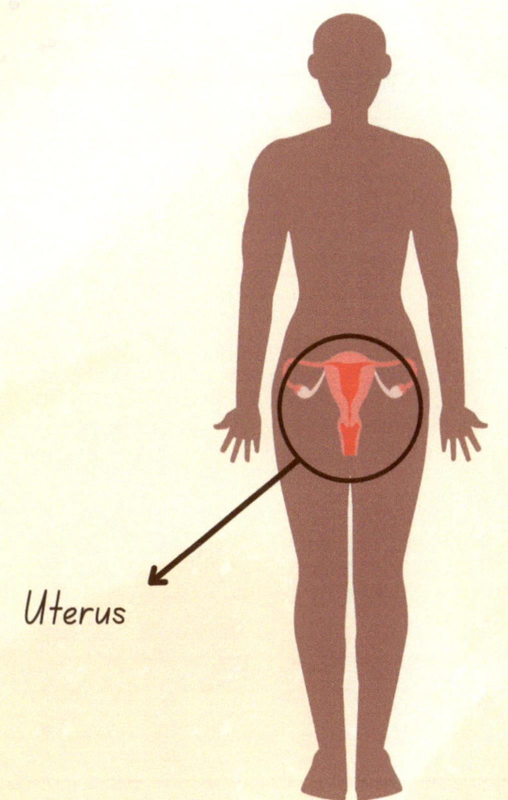

The ovaries are glands
attached to the uterus

They store and release egg cells
during a time in the menstrual cycle
known as ovulation, as well as the
hormones (such as oestrogen and
progesterone) that are responsible
for the menstrual cycle

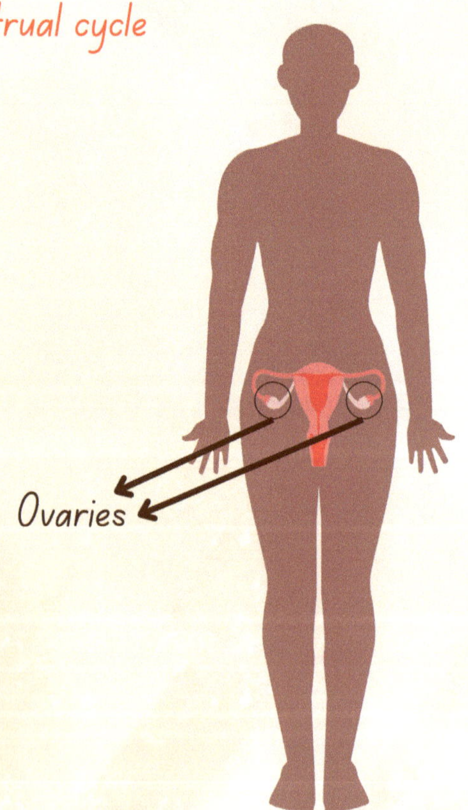

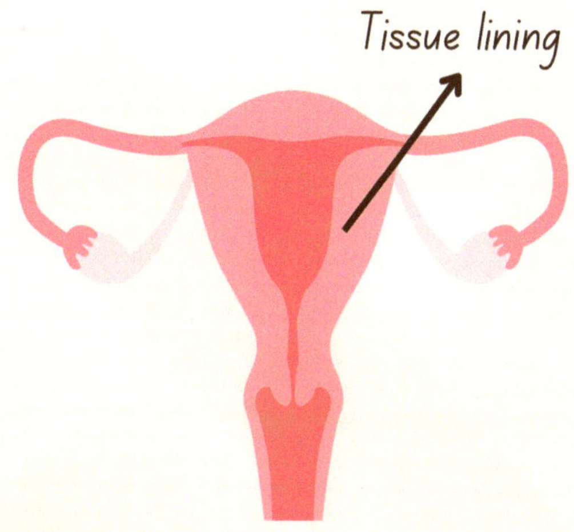

Menstruation is another word
for "having a period" and occurs
when the tissue lining of the
uterus wall breaks down due to
oestrogen and progesterone
levels falling

Oestrogen helps the tissue lining grow while Progesterone helps maintain it throughout most of the menstrual cycle

When these hormones drop during the menstruation period of the cycle, the tissue lining deteriorates

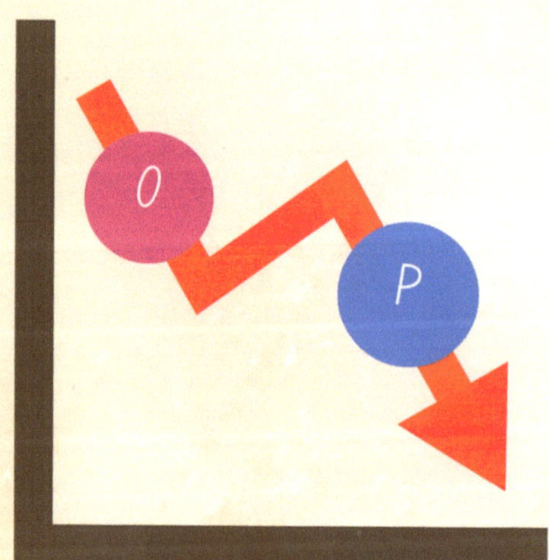

This tissue would have been used in
the development of a baby,
but if the egg cell released by the
ovaries during ovulation isn't fertilised
by a sperm cell and or doesn't
implant onto the lining, it is flushed
out of the body through the vagina

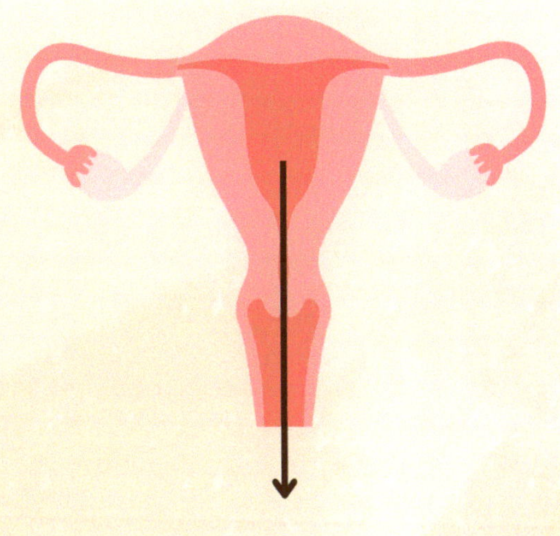

The implantation of a fertilised egg
cell is when it sticks to the thick
tissue lining that has been grown
along the uterus wall

If successful, the implanted egg cell
will progress to form a baby in the
uterus and this will pause
menstruation from taking place

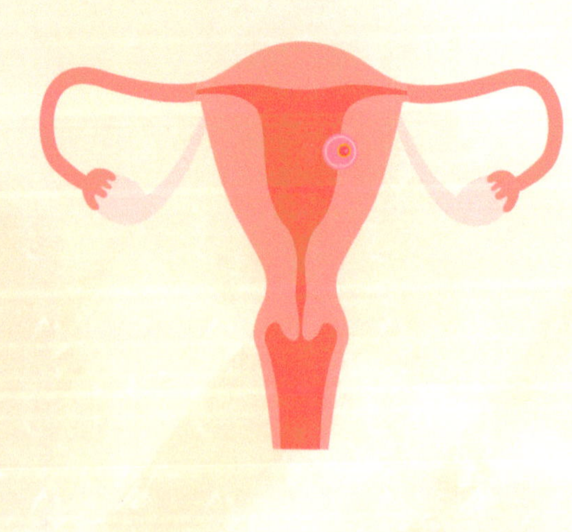

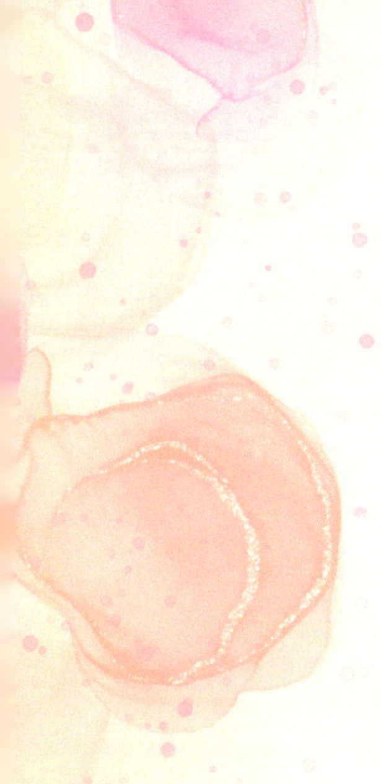

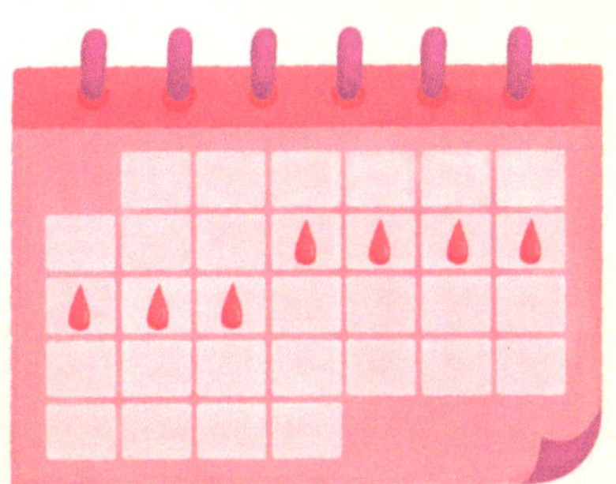

The actual "bleeding through the vagina" lasts 4-8 days, depending on different factors for everyone

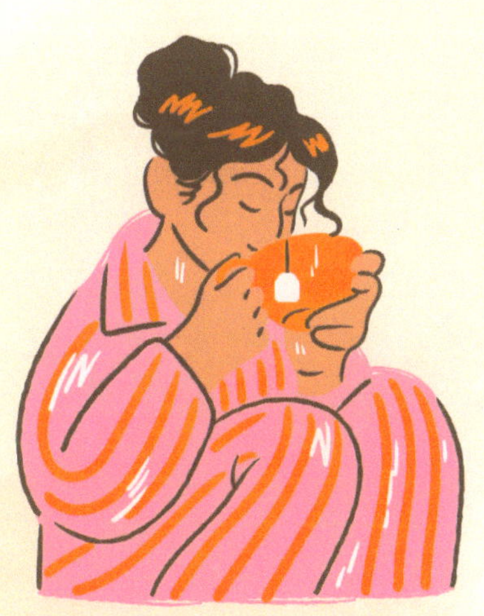

Before a period starts
and or even during, many can
experience PMS or pre-menstrual
symptoms that can heavily impact
their day-to-day lives

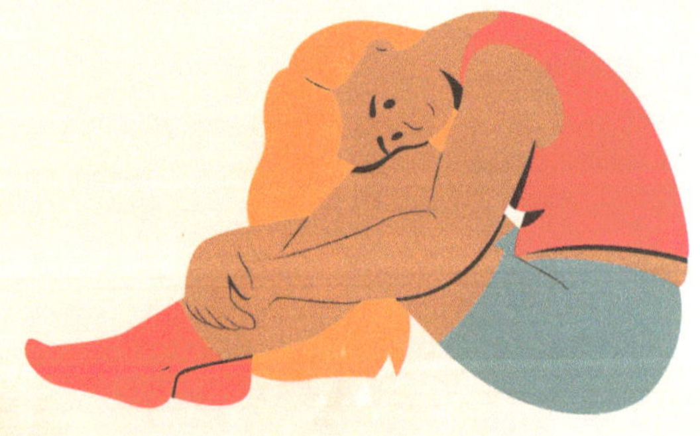

These symptoms can include:

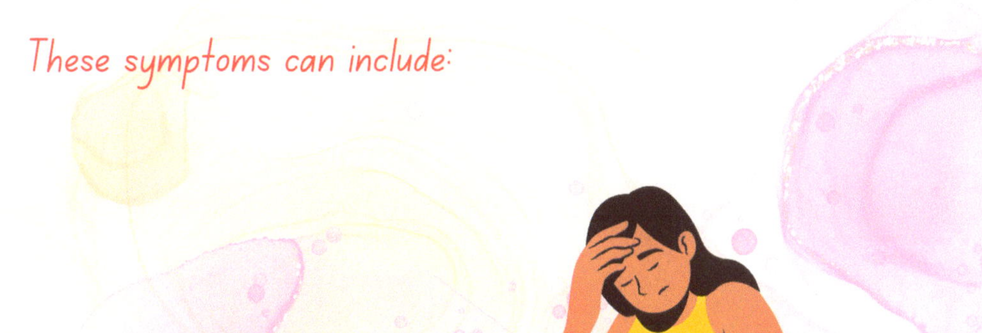

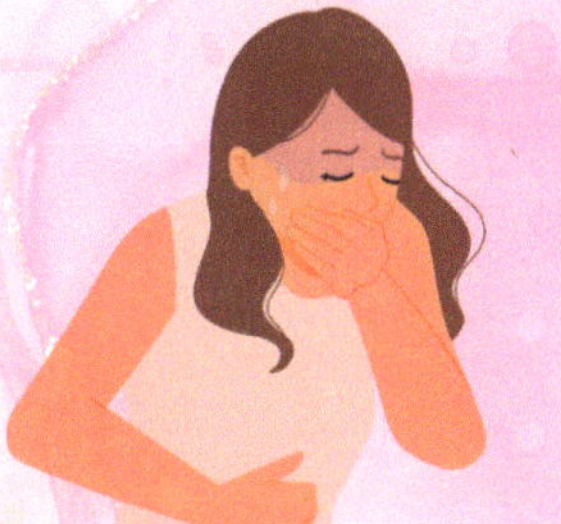

Feeling dizzy
or disoriented

Throwing up, feeling
nauseous and the taste of
food changing

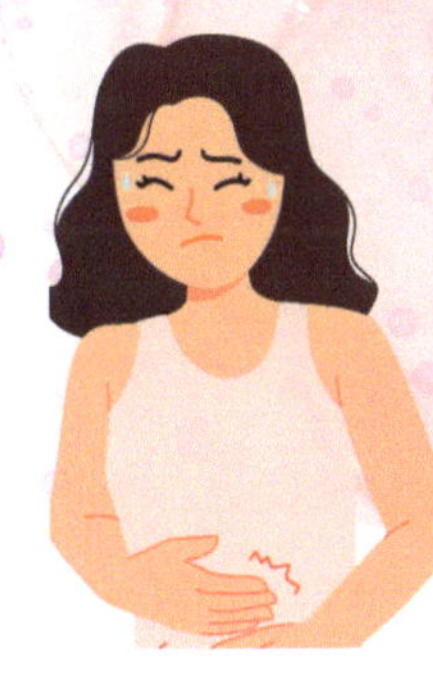

Cramps and

abdominal pain

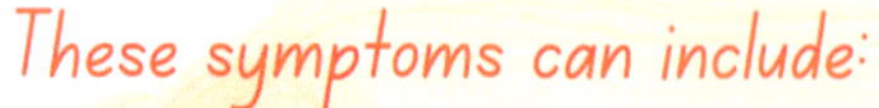

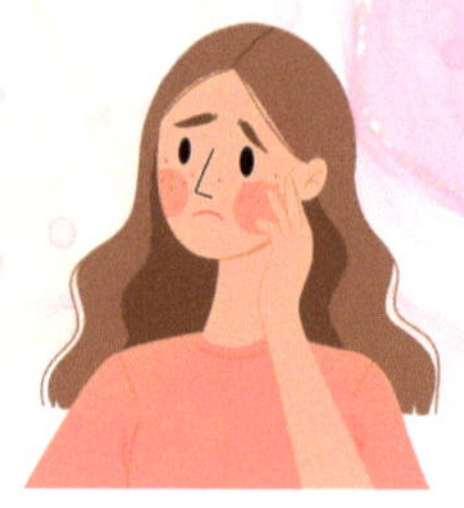

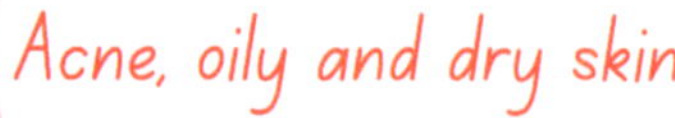

Mood swings that make you
feel frustrated, confused
and tired

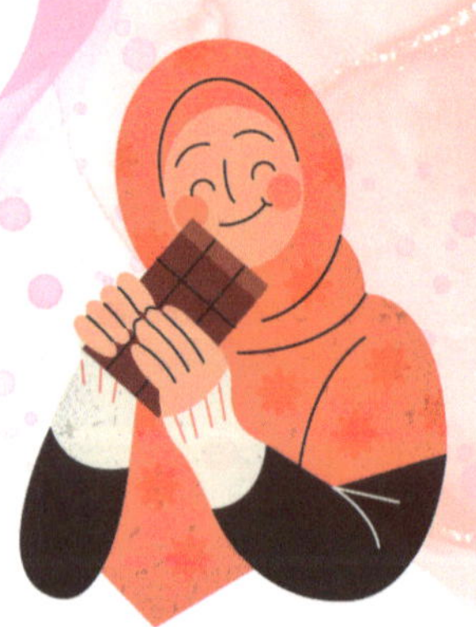

Cravings for specific foods,
such as those high in
sugar and sodium

These symptoms can include:

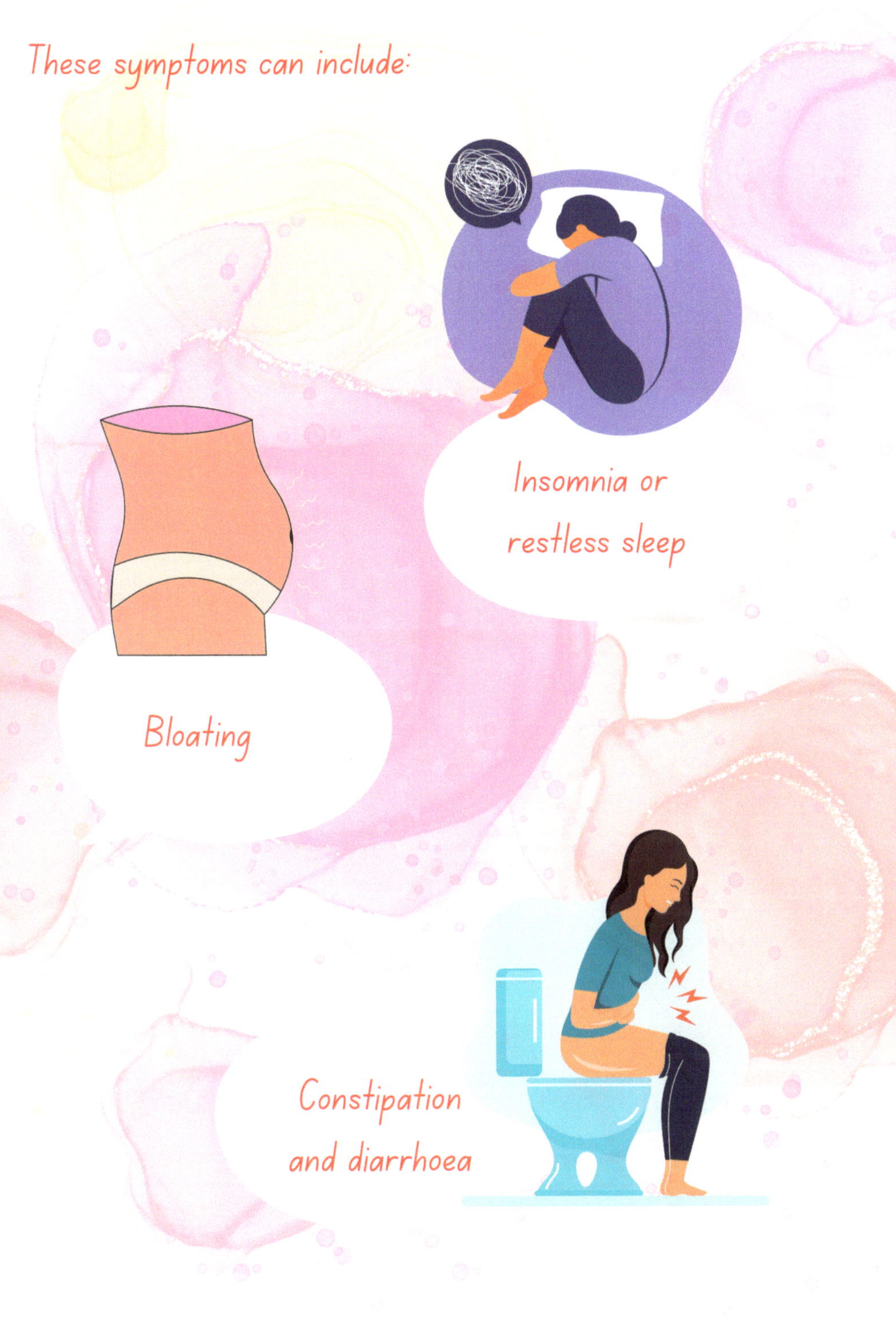

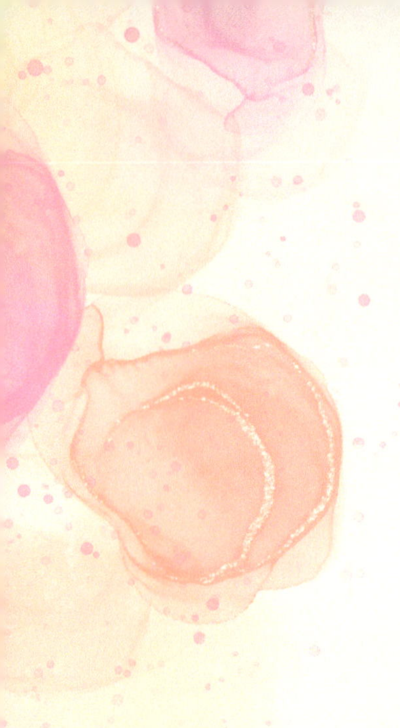

Insomnia can make it very hard to concentrate or complete tasks

Some may feel sluggish and frustrated

Racing thoughts, cold sweats and or cramps can make it difficult to have restful sleep

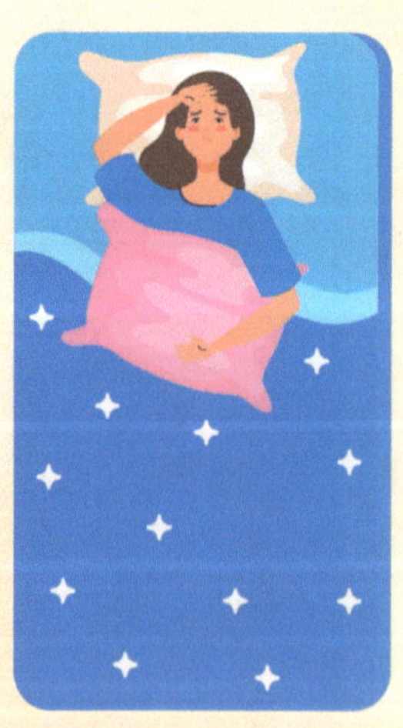

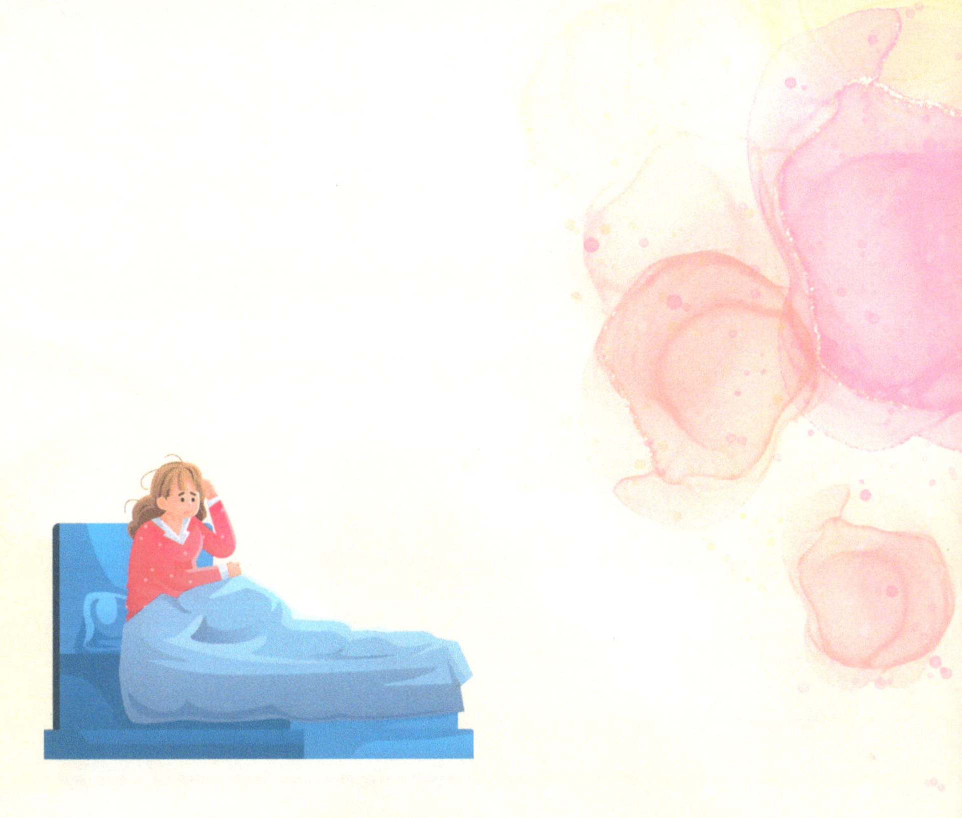

It's okay to wake up feeling awful

A warm drink in the morning and
taking a few minutes to relax the
body before getting started with
the day can make it a little easier

Some may also have
discomfort in and around
their vagina

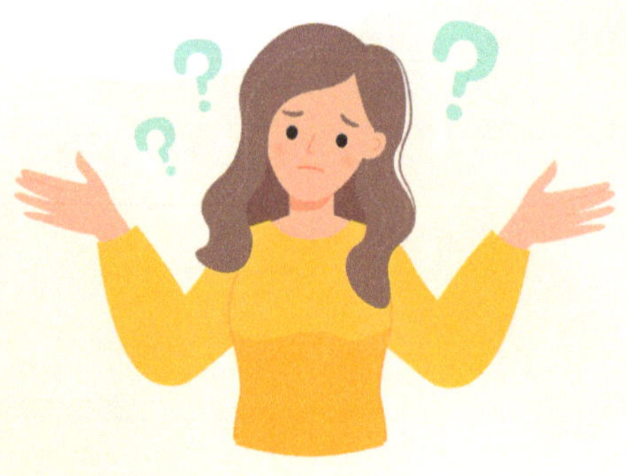

Many hormones spike
and drop rapidly each hour
which can make it very
confusing and uncomfortable

This can be a very stressful time,
so having longer periods of rest
throughout the day can help
reduce the overwhelm

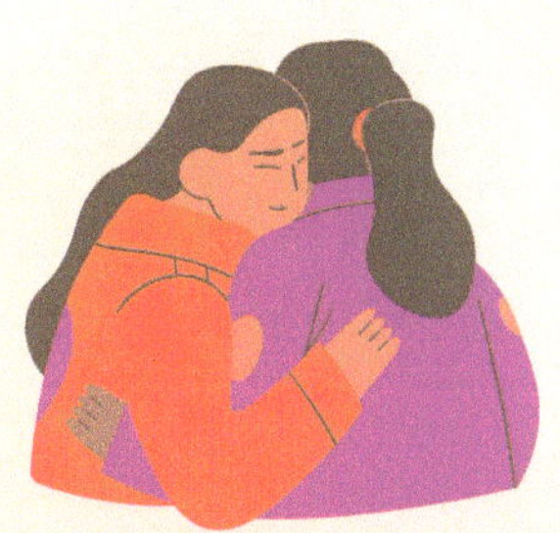

Talking to parents, teachers or
counsellors might help in dealing with
unpleasant emotions

It's okay, feeling isolated
won't last forever

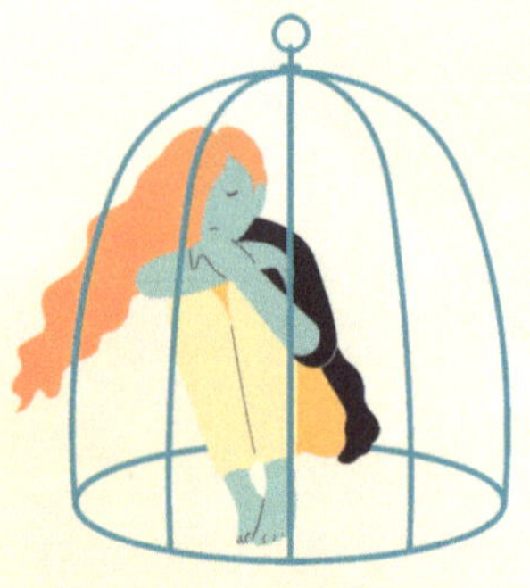

Here are some ways you
can help relieve symptoms
for yourself or a loved one:

Heat packs and hot water
bottles are great for relaxing
muscle pain

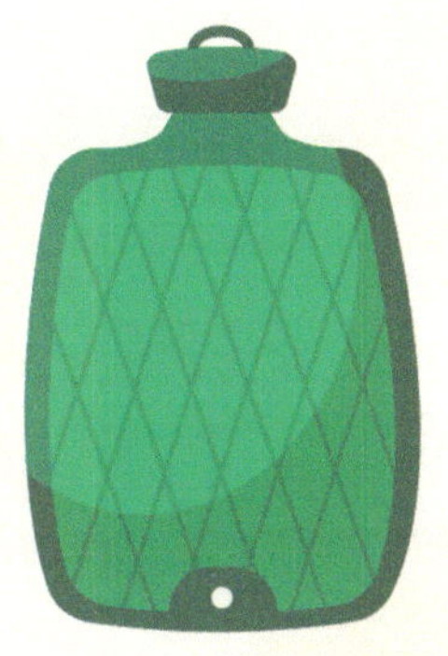

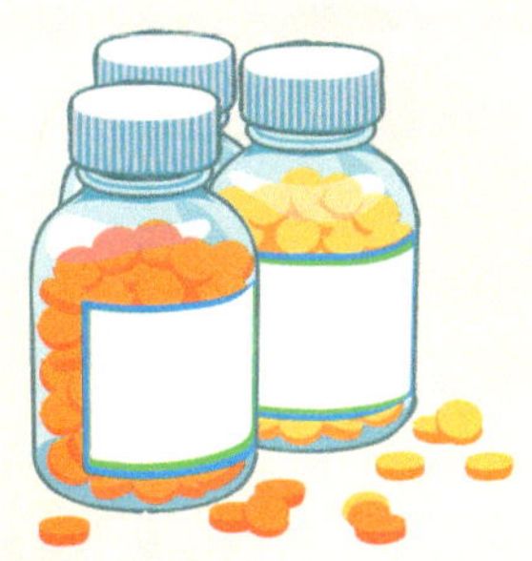

Over-the-counter pain killers
are used for longer-lasting relief

Always check what medication is safe
to use with a GP first as some may
be allergic to certain pain-killers

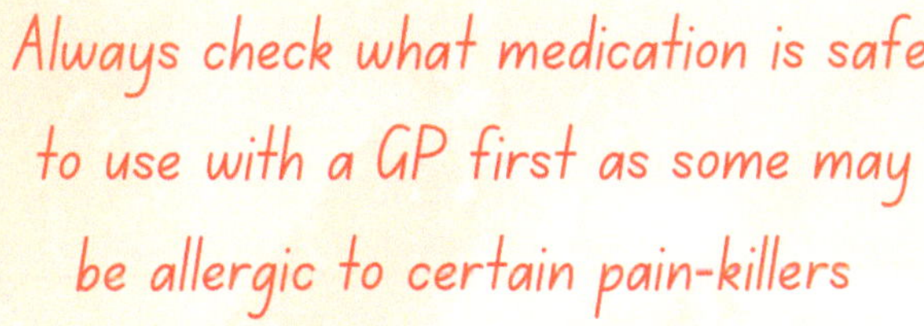

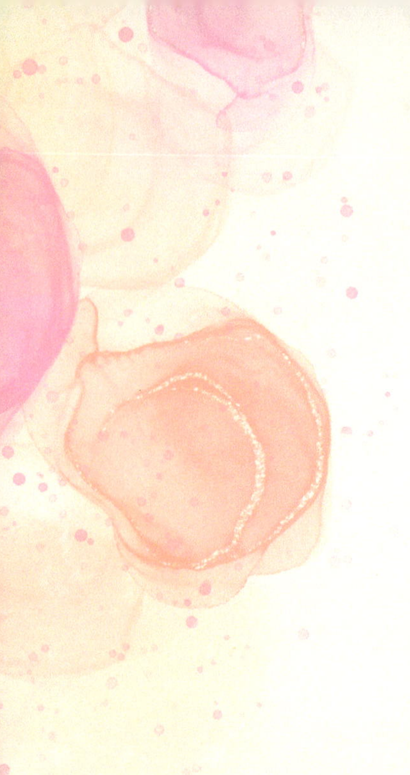

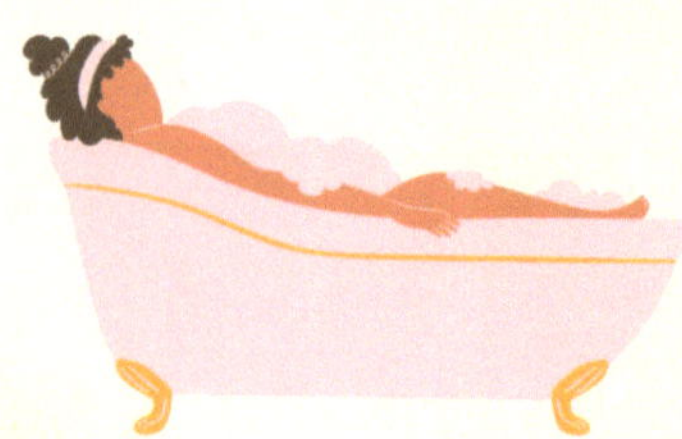

Soaking in an Epsom salt bath
reduces muscle fatigue

Hemp oil/gel/lotion rubbed
below the belly button numbs
muscles around uterus

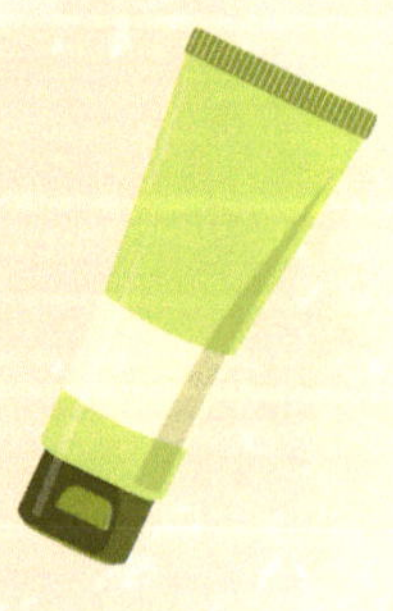

Alternatively, one could journal or log any feelings, thoughts or emotions in a private diary to help sort through them

Writing things down untangles the mind and reduces mental exhaustion

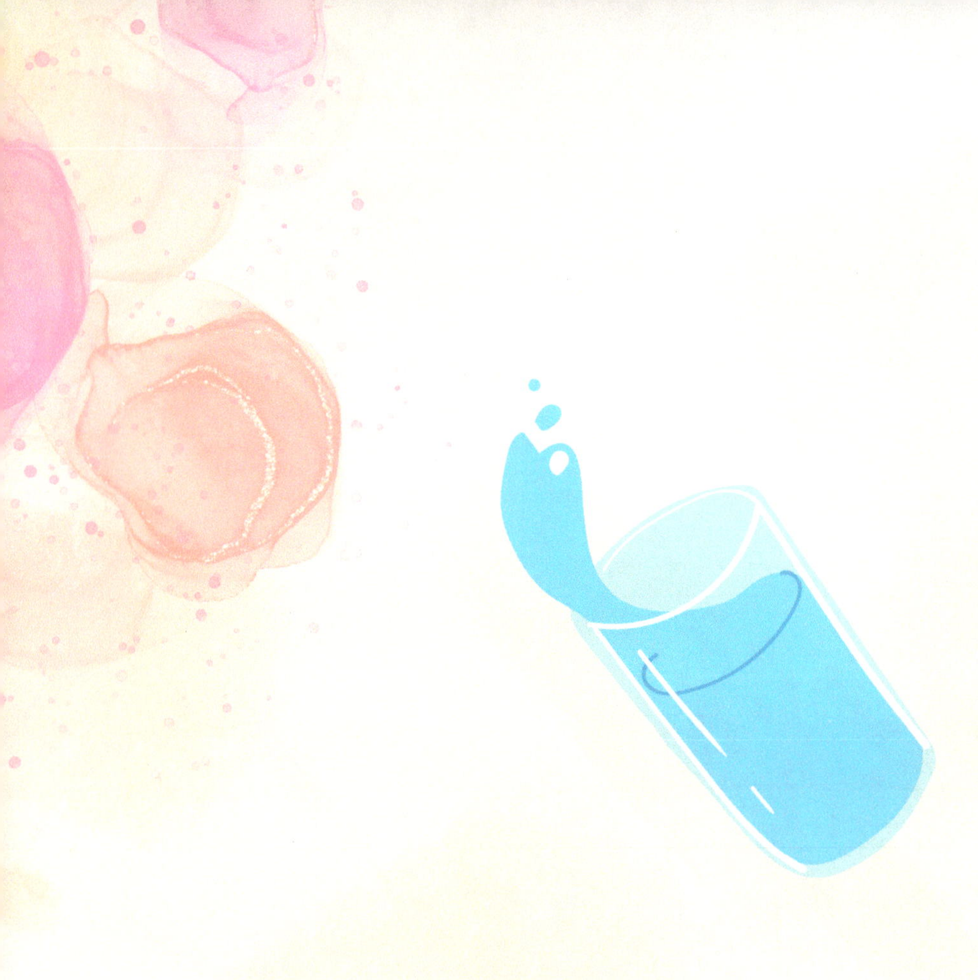

Drinking enough water to stay hydrated
reduces headaches and low moods

It also cools the stomach which can help
with fluctuating appetites

Sometimes, even after
all this care, periods can still
be a little unpredictable

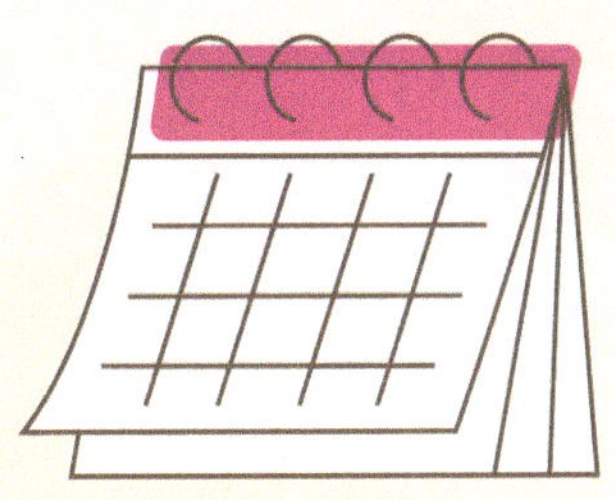

Though a typical menstrual cycle
ranges from 21-35 days, the
menstruation period may not always
be on time every month as this solely
depends on when ovulation occurrs

Periods may be early or late
depending on factors such as stress,
illness, diet or any medication
one may already be on

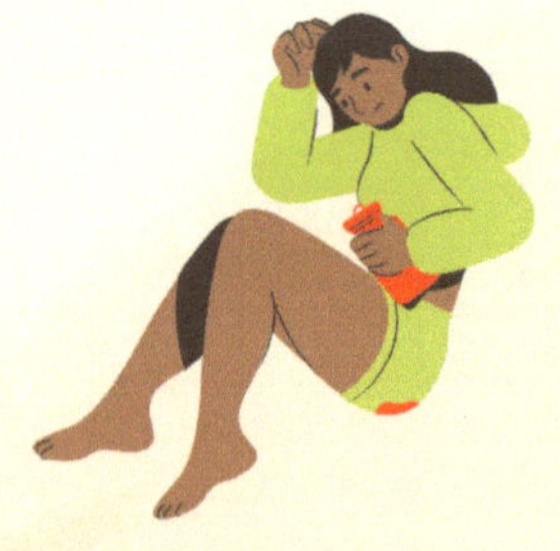 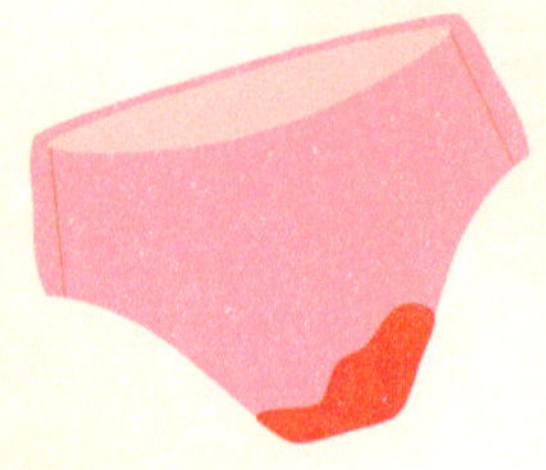

And when it's unexpected, there may
be a few blood stains on clothes!

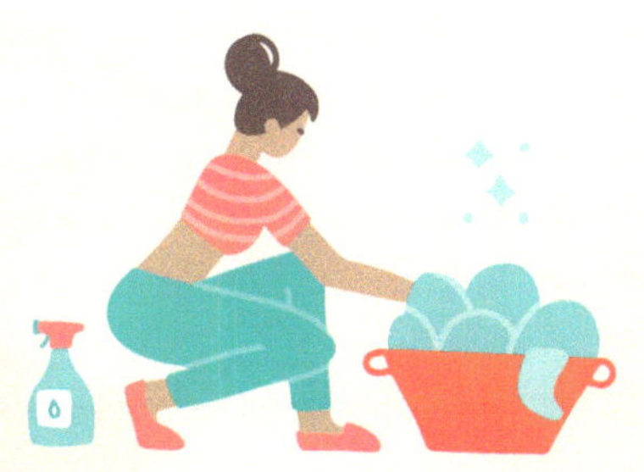

Stain-removers scrubbed over the area
or even just using foaming hand-soap and
scrubbing should be enough to remove
them, even if it takes a little effort

Some hygiene products that
can be used are pads, tampons
or menstrual cups

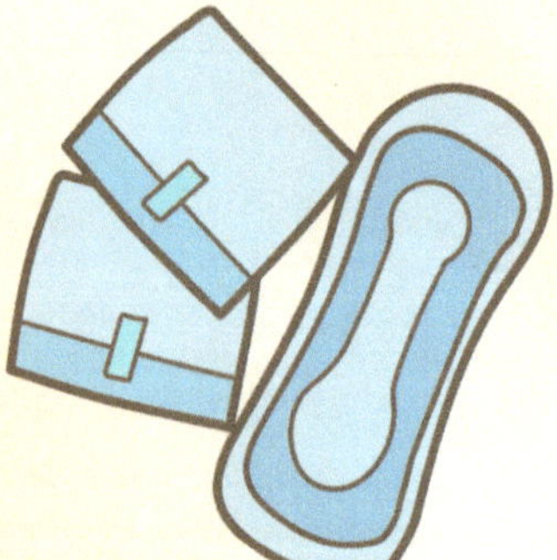

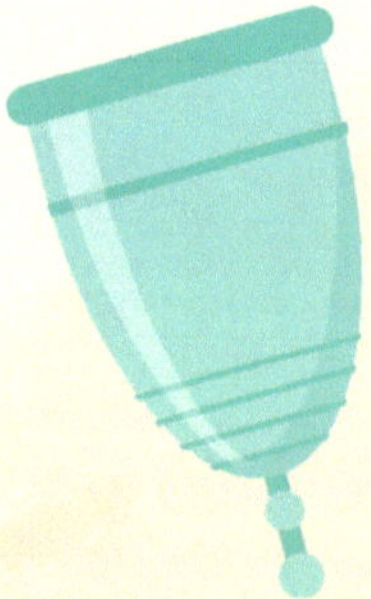

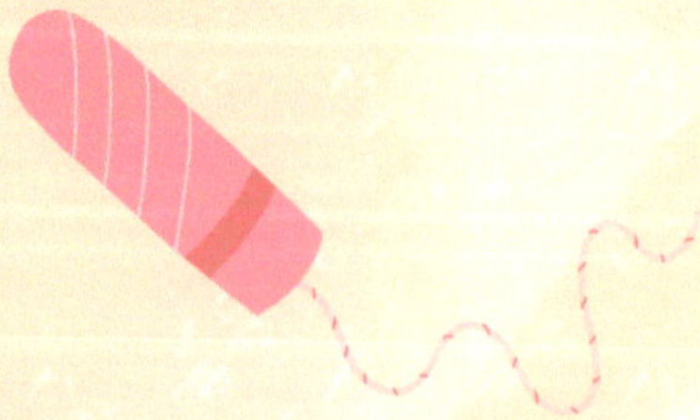

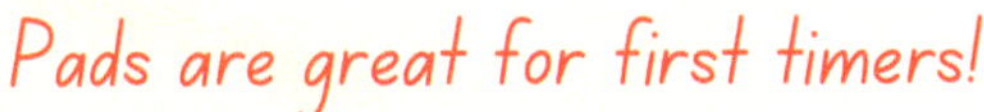

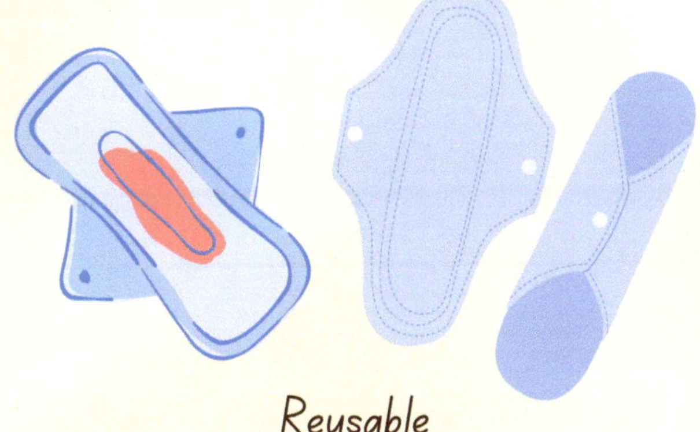

Reusable

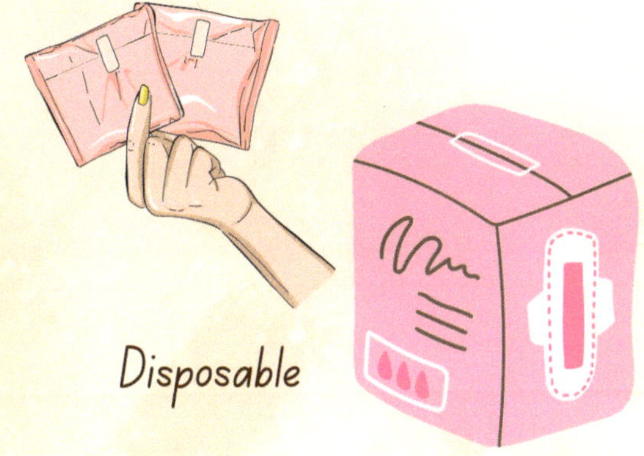

Disposable

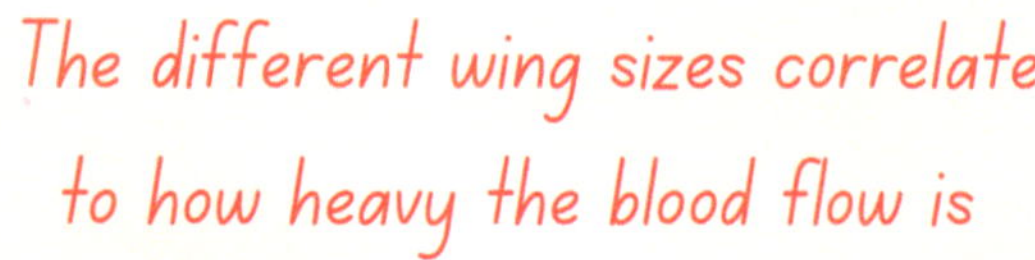

The different wing sizes correlate to how heavy the blood flow is

The bigger the wings, the more blood it can hold

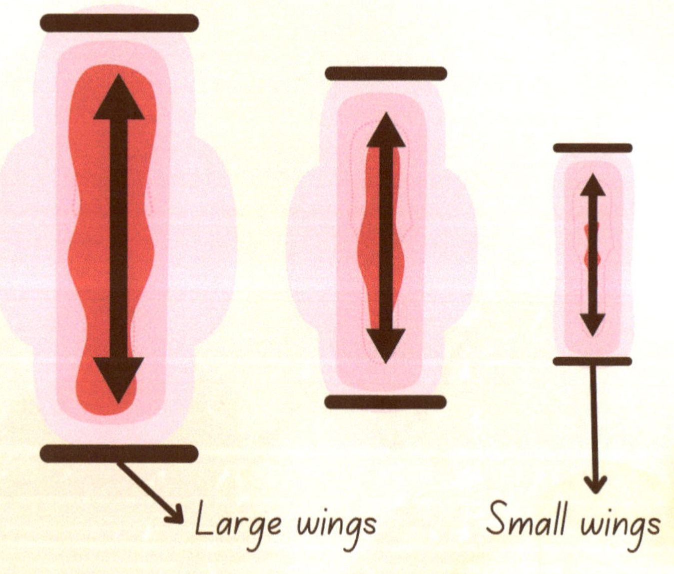

Large wings
Small wings

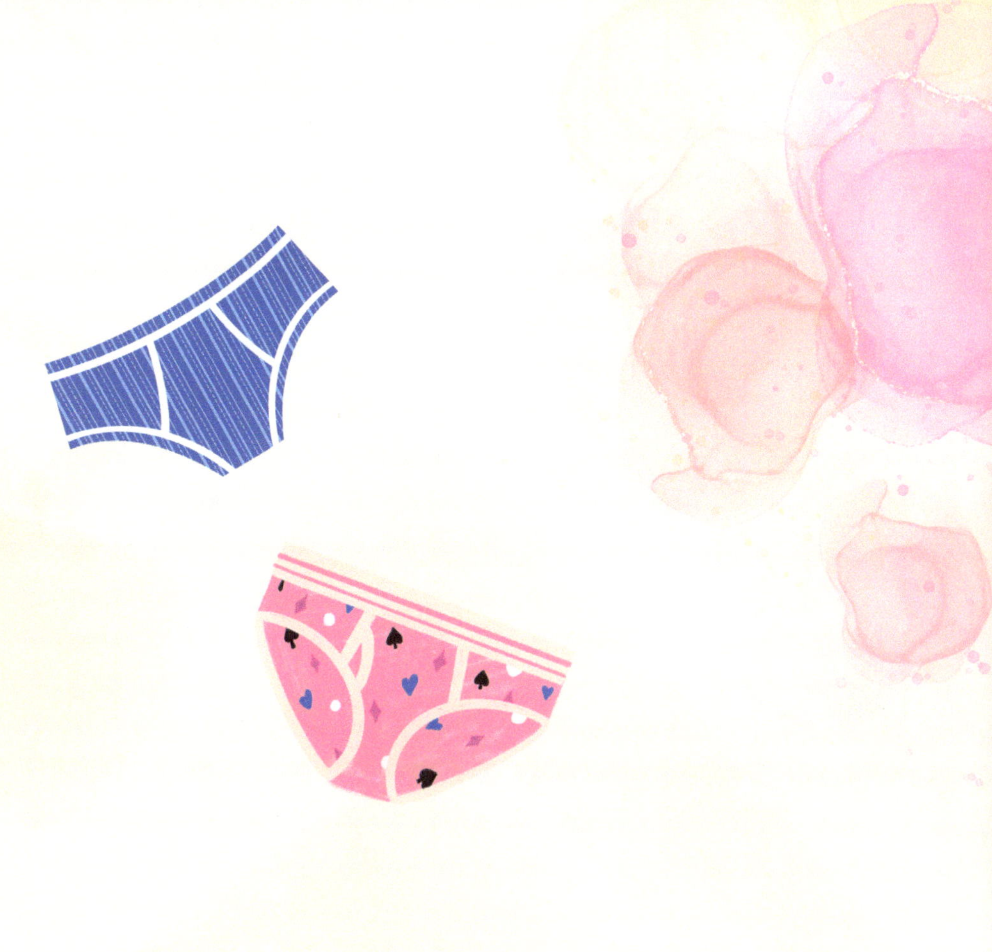

There are also period pants that
have in-built pads and can be worn
as normal clothing

They are machine-washable; just
rinse out the blood after use and put
them in with the dark laundry

Tampons are great if you are
comfortable inserting something
into the vagina but they can take a
little getting used to

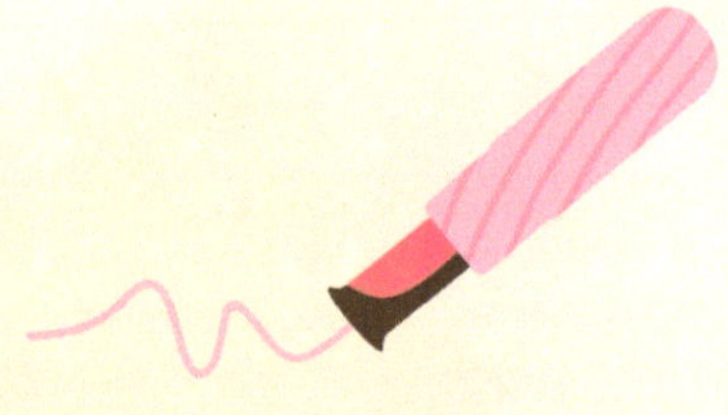

Much like pads, tampon sizes
correspond to the volume of blood
produced during menstruation as
they expand after absorbing it

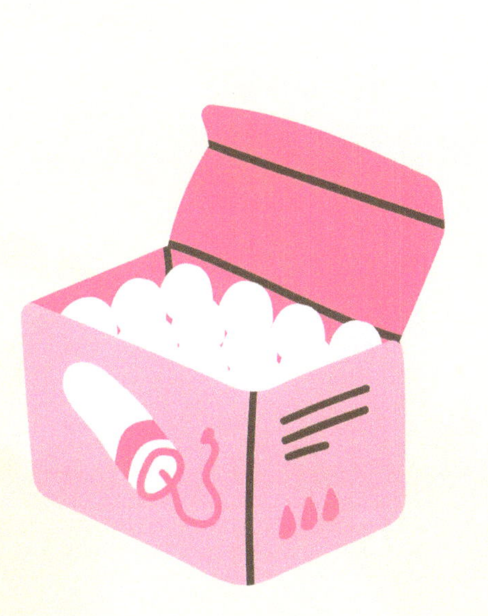

Sizes range from Light to Regular or
Super depending on how heavy a flow is
had, so selecting the right size depends on
the volume of blood produced each day

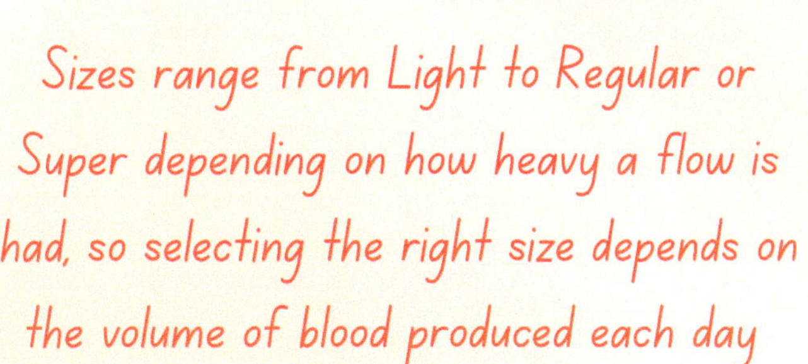

Pulling out a tampon that hasn't
expanded fully can be a little painful,
otherwise, due to friction against the
vaginal wall

To insert a tampon into the vagina, hold it at a 45° angle towards the ground before pushing it all the way in, leaving the string so that it can be pulled out again

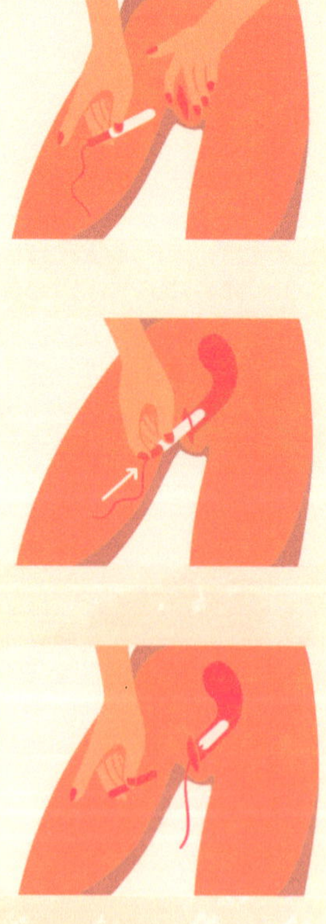

Tampons can also come with an
applicator that has a smooth
surface to reduce friction and
can make it easier to insert

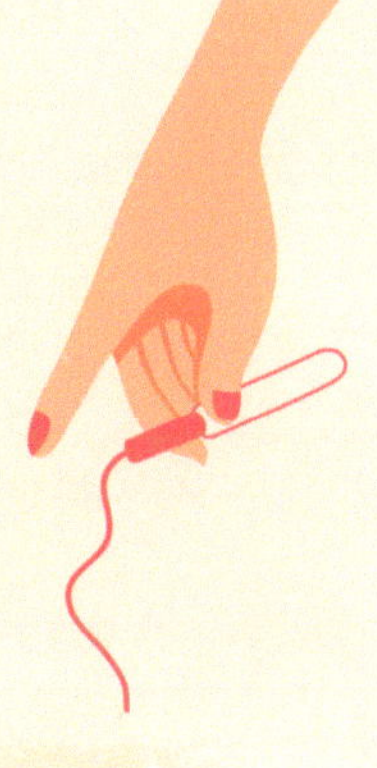

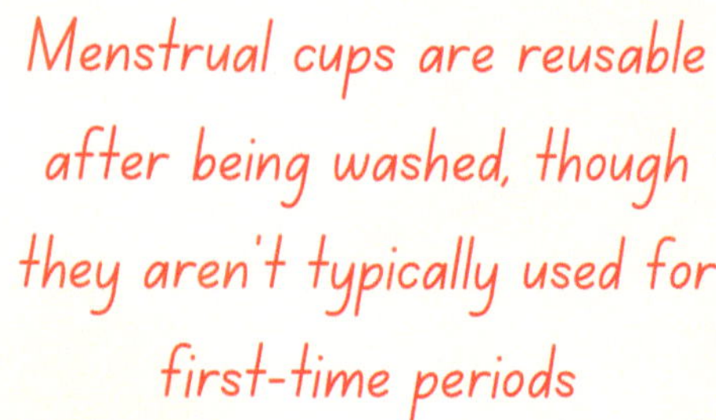

Menstrual cups are reusable after being washed, though they aren't typically used for first-time periods

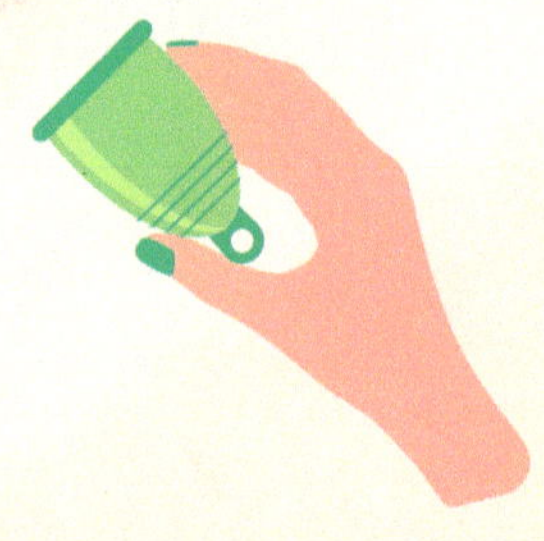

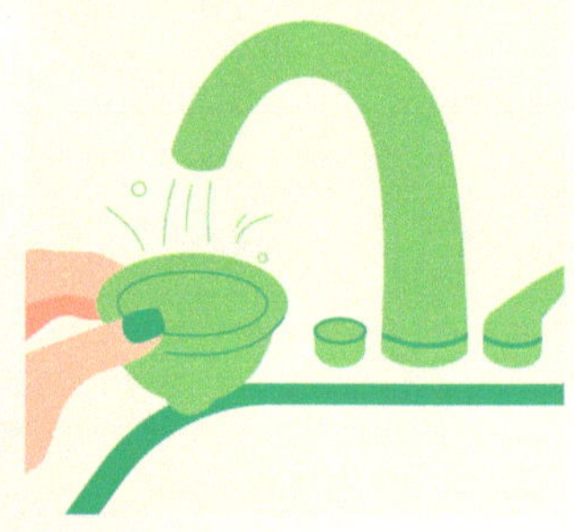

They are silicon cups that collect the blood once inserted into the vagina and then need to be removed, emptied and washed before use again

Instructions on how to wear them and some of the potential risks are included on the box, which is why they are typically used by older woman

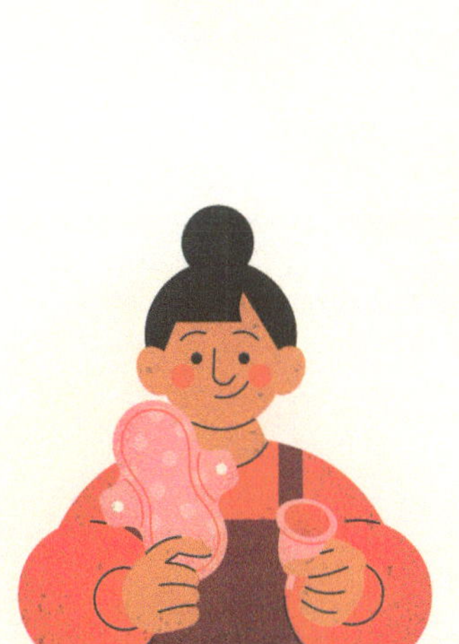

However, like reusable pads, they are a more environmentally friendly option and are less costly long-term

To insert a cup, fold it in half and gently rotate it into the vagina so that it opens up once inside

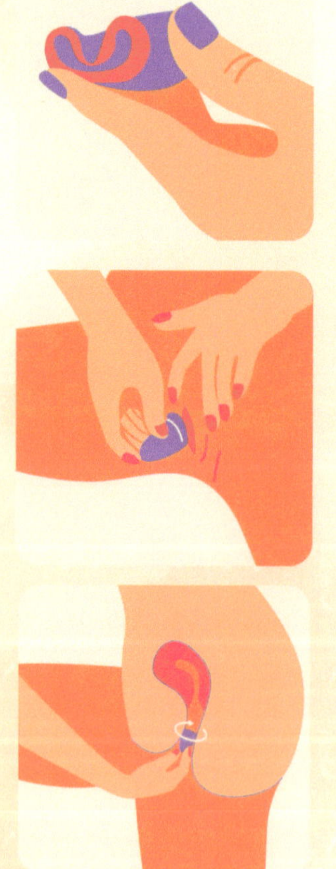

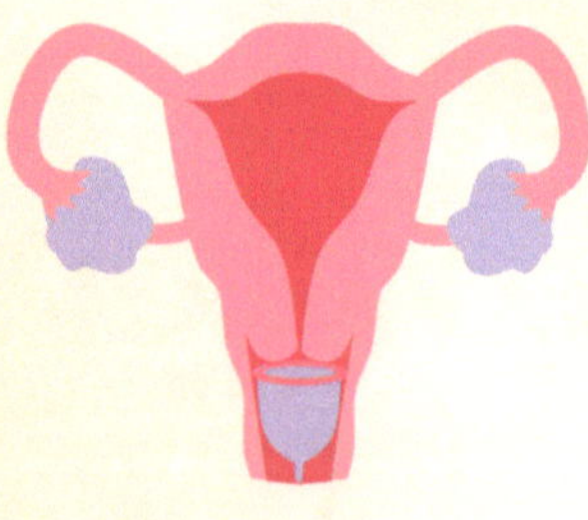

If you are experiencing menstruation,
there are no rules

You can use whatever feels the best
for you and gives you the best
support during your period

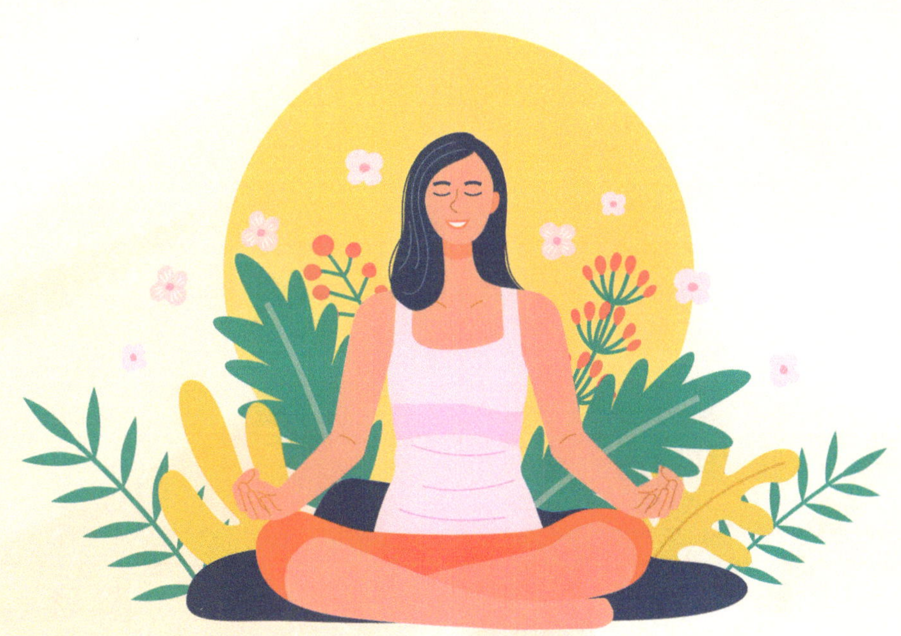

Author's Note:

Thank you so much for purchasing my book!
If you liked this book, please consider leaving a
review and recommending it to someone who
would be interested in learning about periods.

For more information, reach me through...

Email: pitayapages@gmail.com
Instagram: @pitayapages
Ko-Fi: pitayapages